ARE YOU SWEET ENOUGH

ALREADY?

ARE YOU SWEET ENOUGH ALREADY?

Top 10 Low Glycemic Load Desserts

For Blood Sugar Control

Includes a Handy Bonus Guide for Creating Your Own Delicious Low Glycemic Load Recipes

By

Judith Lickus B. Sc., LBSW

Published for

Diabetes Manager

Corpus Christi, TX 78463

Notice

Glycemic Index scores used in the calculations for the recipes are from the International Tables of Glycemic Index and Glycemic Load Values: 2008, published by the US National Library of Medicine National Institutes of Health. Carbohydrate content is from the USDA National Nutrient Database for Standard Reference.

In 2013, a precedent setting meeting of international nutrition experts convened on a little island off the coast of Italy. The outcome of their meeting was a consensus statement proclaiming that "The Glycemic Load (GL) is the single best predictor of the glycemic response."

The recipes in this book rest on the foundation of that precedent setting proclamation. They are *justified* by delivering a low glycemic load score for each serving, as defined by the consensus committee to be 10 or less.

This book is sold with the understanding that the author is not liable for the misconception or misuse of any information provided. The information presented here is in no way intended as a substitute for medical treatment or nutritional counseling.

ISBN-13: 978-152303996
ISBN-10: 1523803391

DEDICATION

This book is dedicated exclusively to those individuals who believe that numbers really do count.

Whether you are someone who prefers to know the nutritional values in the food you eat, or you have to monitor your blood sugar levels as a necessity, you recognize the power of the *absolute* nature of mathematics over the *relative* nature of our humanity.

This difference sets you apart from the majority.

If you are looking for delicious, satisfying, decadent desserts that won't throw your numbers off, this book is a great start.

For you, we present the 10 top Decadent Low Glycemic Load Dessert Contest Winners to tickle your palate and keep those important numbers right where you want them.

INTRODUCTION

The World Health Organization favors the use of the glycemic index (GI) and glycemic load (GL) tools for natural blood glucose control.

But when people start to use these tools, drug companies and food product manufacturers see a decrease in their corporate profits. So there is no advertising for these food facts.

This makes getting the word out to others difficult. That's because individuals and families are the only ones who benefit. So our health becomes a matter of self-responsibility. But at least we know the truth.

Sure, we can ask our doctors about these tools. But many health professionals consider the glycemic index and glycemic load to be too complex and too variable to use in their busy practice. So we have to figure out how to use these tools for ourselves. We have to help each other.

SELF DETERMINATION

We believe that each individual has the right to judge these tools for him or herself. But first, let's see if you've got what it takes:

1. Did you learn arithmetic in the 5th grade?
2. Are you willing to take some time to help yourself?
3. Would you like to eliminate diabetic complications, medications and the side-effects they can cause?

It's not your fault that you got in this situation. But it is up to you whether you stay or not.

Your body is the greatest miracle in the world. Bless your beautiful body with natural, health building wholesome foods. You have to help get the word out to others.

This is a little quick-start guide that brings you some tasty recipes. Then it brings you to the very best resources and walks you through how to use them.

Whether your kitchen uses the Metric System or US Legal Measures, we've got you covered.

DESSERTS THAT BUILD HEALTH

- The recipes in this book will help you get off to a good start. Every one of them shows you the *glycemic index* and the *low glycemic load* score + other nutrition details for each serving. You don't have to suffer with blood sugar swings over a few moments of pleasure anymore -- and you can skip the side serving of guilt or shame.
- All of these recipes are low in carbs and free of wheat and grains. There are recipes for every taste. All of the recipes come with easy-to-follow directions.
- The *Special Bonus Section* teaches you how you can use the Glycemic Index and Glycemic Load. It also puts you in touch with the best resources to use for

creating your own low glycemic load recipes and meals.

We start with natural, unprocessed whole foods. You might be surprised to find that the only ingredient that comes out of a box is a little bit of baking soda. Low glycemic sweeteners such as stevia and coconut palm sugar provide sweetening.

None of these recipes contain any of the other over 50 deceptive names for "sugar" commonly used in products today. Those are the misleading names for sugar that serve to "hook" you into sugar addiction – even if you are a "label reader" already. And that addiction is what causes the cravings that can make your sweet tooth go wild.

You will see how easy it is to leave sugar addiction behind. And you can get started by enjoying some healthful, decadently delicious, low glycemic load desserts.

❧TABLE OF CONTENTS ❧

RANGER COOKIES

YIELD: 24 cookies serve 12
Per portion:

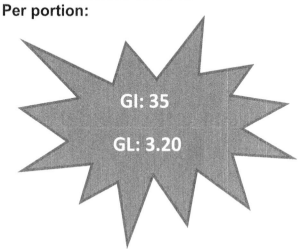

GI: 35

GL: 3.20

CALORIES: 202; Carbohydrates: 9.16g; Fiber: 10.25g; Protein: 4.73g; Fat: 18.27g; Saturated Fats: 5.82g; Sodium: 58mg

INGREDIENTS:
- 1 ½ cups (360 mL) ground almonds or almond meal flour
- 2 oz. (59 mL) unsalted butter (preferably organic)
- 2 oz. (59 mL) coconut oil
- 3 Tbsp. (44 mL) coconut palm sugar
- 1 egg
- 1 oz. (30 mL) cocoa nibs
- 1 oz. (30 mL) pecan halves
- 1 Tbsp. (15 mL) cinnamon
- 1 tsp. (5 mL) vanilla extract

- 1 tsp. (5 mL) almond extract
- ½ tsp. (2 mL) baking soda
- 1 pinch of sea salt

PREPARATION:

1. Preheat oven to 350° F (177° C).
2. Over very low heat, melt butter and coconut oil, and mix well.
3. In a small mixing bowl, beat egg well.
4. Add vanilla and almond extracts, coconut palm sugar, and mix well.
5. In a large mixing bowl, combine almond meal flour (breaking up any lumps), baking soda, and salt. Set aside.
6. Add egg to coconut oil mixture, mixing very well.
7. Pour liquid mixture into almond meal flour mixture, stirring very well.
8. Form dough into tsp. sized cookies.
9. Flatten the top of each cookie with a half pecan pressed into the middle of each cookie.
10. Place them on a baking sheet and bake for 8-10 minutes.

PUMPKIN CUSTARD

YIELD: Serves 8
Per portion:

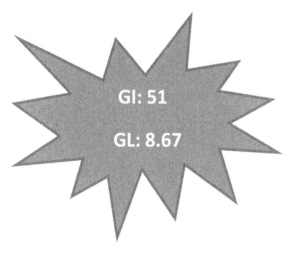

GI: 51

GL: 8.67

CALORIES: 123; Carbohydrates: 17g; Fiber: 1.71g;
Protein: 5.53g; Fat: 5.08g; Saturated Fats: 2.75g;
Sodium: 74.12mg

INGREDIENTS:
- One 15 oz. (425 g) can 100% pure pumpkin
- One 14 oz. (354 mL) can evaporated milk
- 2 large eggs
- 1 Tbsp. (15 mL) unsalted organic butter
- 1 tsp. (5 mL) cinnamon
- ½ tsp. (2 mL) organic vanilla extract
- Liquid Stevia to taste, optional

TOPPING (OPTIONAL):
- 8 tsp. (39 mL) sugar-free whipped topping
- 8 sprinkles of cinnamon

PREPARATION:
1. Preheat oven to 325° F (163° C).
2. Coat the cooking surface of a 9 X 2 inch (23 X 4 cm) glass baking dish with butter.
3. In a large mixing bowl, beat eggs well; add vanilla, stevia, and cinnamon. Combine thoroughly.
4. Add canned pumpkin to egg mixture, combining well.
5. Add evaporated milk to pumpkin mixture, being sure to combine very well.
6. Pour pumpkin mixture into buttered baking dish and place in center of oven.
7. Bake for about 45 minutes, or until knife inserted into center comes out clean.
8. Remove baking dish of custard to a cloth covered wire rack to cool. Refrigerate overnight before serving.
9. Top each serving with 1 tsp. (5 mL) of sugar-free whipped topping and a sprinkle of cinnamon.

CHOCOLADO PARFAITS

YIELD: Serves 2
Per portion:

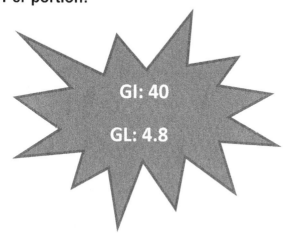

GI: 40

GL: 4.8

CALORIES: 130; Carbohydrates: 12g; Fiber: 5.65g; Protein: 1g; Fat: 9.17g; Saturated Fats: 1.66g; Sodium: 9mg

INGREDIENTS:
- 2 small ripe avocados, ½ cup (120 mL) pureed
- 2 Tbsp. (30 mL) unsweetened cocoa powder
- 2 packets stevia
- 1 tsp. (5 mL) dry instant coffee crystals
- ½ tsp. (2 mL) organic vanilla extract
- ½ tsp. (2 mL) almond extract
- 4 Tbsp. (59 mL) sugar-free whipped topping
- 2 fresh cherries, strawberies, or rasberries

PREPARATION:

1. Slice avocados in half, lengthwise, all the way around the seed. Separate halves and squeeze to remove seeds.
2. Scrape avocado meat from shell into a medium-sized mixing bowl.
3. Using an electric beater or mashing very thoroughly with a fork, cream avocado until very smooth.
4. In a small bowl, combine cocoa, coffee crystals and stevia well.
5. Add cocoa mixture to avocado mixture. Scrape sides of bowl with a bowl scraper frequently to incorporate all of avocado, cocoa, sweetener and extracts.
6. Blend very well until smooth and creamy.
7. Spoon alternately into parfait glasses, layering with a spoonful of Whipped topping.
8. Garnish each parfait with a cherry or raspberry.
9. Freeze for about 30 minutes before serving.

BROWNIE BISCOTTIES

YIELD: Serves 12
Per portion:

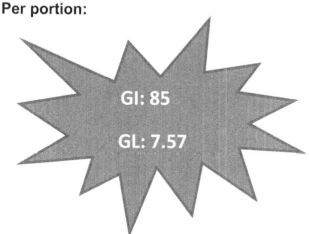

GI: 85

GL: 7.57

CALORIES: 106.57; Carbohydrates: 8.90g; Fiber: 1.28g; Protein: 2.94g; Fat: 8.3g; Saturated Fats: 5.58g; Sodium: 53.78mg

INGREDIENTS:
- ½ cup (120 mL) butter, melted
- ½ cup (120 mL) unsweetened cocoa powder
- ½ cup (120 mL) coconut palm sugar
- 2 eggs
- 5 tsp. (25 mL) arrowroot powder
- ½ tsp. (2 mL) aluminum free baking powder
- ¼ tsp. (1 mL) salt
- 1 tsp. (5 mL) organic vanilla extract
- 1 tsp. (5 mL) organic almond extract

PREPARATION:
1. Preheat oven to 350° F (177° C).
2. Beat all ingredients together very well with an electric mixer in a medium sized mixing bowl.
3. Pour into 8 X 9 inch (20 X 23 cm) glass baking dish.
4. Bake for 20 – 25 minutes until wooden pick inserted in center comes out clean.
5. Cool on a wire rack or trivet covered with a soft cloth.
6. Slice into 12 long strips.
7. Slice again through center of baking dish, creating 24 crispy brownie strips so that everyone can have two on their plate.

GINGERBREAD BABY-CAKES

YIELD: Serves 12
Per portion:

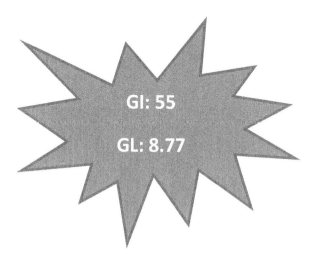

GI: 55

GL: 8.77

CALORIES: 81.47; Carbohydrates: 15.94g; Fiber: 1.67g; Protein: 3.35g; Fat: 9.32g; Saturated Fats: 3.33g; Sodium: 138.10mg

INGREDIENTS:
- 1 ¼ cup (300 mL) almond meal flour, twice sifted
- ¼ cup (60 mL) coconut flour
- ¾ cup (180 mL) water
- 1 extra-large egg
- ½ cup (120 mL) coconut palm sugar
- 1/3 cup (80 mL) coconut oil
- ½ cup (120 mL) blackstrap molasses
- 1 tsp. (5 mL) ginger
- ½ tsp. (2 mL) baking soda

- ¼ tsp. (1 mL) salt

PREPARATION:
1. Preheat oven to 350° F (177° C).
2. Combine coconut oil and sugar in a medium sized mixing bowl. Beat with an electric mixer until creamy and smooth. Add egg, and mix thoroughly.
3. In a separate bowl combine water and molasses.
4. In another bowl, mix almond meal flour, coconut flour, baking soda, salt, and ginger.
5. Add molasses and dry ingredients alternately to sugar mixture, combining thoroughly after each addition.
6. Distribute mixture evenly among a non-stick cupcake baking sheet with a capacity of 12.
7. Bake in pre-heated oven for 28 to 32 minutes, until wooden pick inserted in center of a cupcake comes out clean.

CHOCOLATE AVOCADO CREAM PIE

YIELD: 12 servings
Per portion:

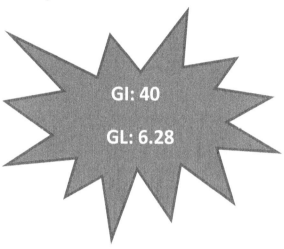

GI: 40

GL: 6.28

CALORIES: 312; Carbohydrates: 15.69g; Fiber: 9.32g; Protein: 10.86g; Fat: 28.42g; Saturated Fats: 5.29g; Sodium: 6.3mg

INGREDIENTS FOR CRUST:
- 1 cup (240 mL) ground pecans
- ½ cup (120 mL) almond meal
- ½ cup (120 mL) flax meal
- 2 Tbsp. (30 mL) unsweetened cocoa powder
- 2 packets stevia
- 4 Tbsp. (59 mL) organic coconut oil
- 1 Tbsp. (15 mL) unsalted organic butter

INGREDIENTS FOR FILLING:
- 5 large ripe avocados, 2 cups (480 mL) pureed

- 6 Tbsp. (89 mL) cocoa
- 9 packets stevia
- 1 Tbsp. (15 mL) dry instant coffee crystals
- 1 tsp. (5 mL) organic vanilla extract
- 1 tsp. (5 mL) almond extract
- 1 cup (240 mL) fresh cherries, strawberries, or raspberries, rinsed and gently patted dry

PREPARATION:

For Crust:
1. Melt butter and coconut oil over low heat in a medium sized stainless steel bowl.
2. Combine ground pecans, almond meal, flax meal, cocoa, and stevia in a small bowl.
3. Add combined nut mixture to melted butter and coconut oil mixture. Mix well until thoroughly combined.
4. Press mixture into a 9 inch (23 X 4 cm) round pie dish to form a crust.)

For Filling:
1. Slice avocados in half, lengthwise, all the way around the seed. Separate halves and squeeze to remove seeds.
2. Scrape avocado meat from shell into a medium-sized mixing bowl.
3. Using an electric beater or mashing very thoroughly with a fork, cream avocado until very smooth.
4. In a small bowl, combine cocoa, coffee crystals and stevia well.
5. Add cocoa mixture to avocado mixture. Scrape sides of bowl with a bowl scraper

frequently to incorporate all of avocado,
cocoa, sweetener and extracts.

6.   Blend very well until smooth and creamy and
       scoop into pie crust.

7.   Garnish with a circle of beautiful fresh
       cherries, strawberries, or raspberries.

8.   Refrigerate until ready to serve.

PINA COLADA UP-SIDE-DOWN CAKE

YIELD: Serves 16
Per portion:

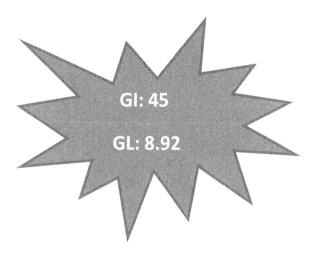

GI: 45

GL: 8.92

CALORIES: 126; Carbohydrates: 19.83g; Fiber: 2.94g; Protein: 5.26g; Fat: 5g; Saturated Fats: 3.15g; Sodium: 114mg

INGREDIENTS:
- One 20 ounce (567 g) can sliced pineapple
- One 16 ounce (454 g) can butter beans, drained
- 6 eggs
- 1/4 cup (60 mL) coconut oil, melted
- 1/3 cup (80 mL) coconut palm sugar
- 1 Tbsp. (15 mL) coconut palm sugar
- 1/3 cup (80 mL) coconut flour
- 1 ½ tsp. (7 mL) aluminum free baking powder
- 1 tsp. (5 mL) baking soda
- 1 tsp. (5 mL) organic vanilla extract

- 12 pecan halves
- 1 Tbsp. (15 mL) unsalted organic butter
- 8 tsp. (39 mL) sugar-free whipped topping, if desired

PREPARATION:
1.   Preheat oven to 325° F (163° C).
2.   Melt butter over very low heat in 9 inch (23 X 4 cm) round glass baking dish, being careful to coat cooking surface with butter. Sprinkle 1 Tbsp. (15 mL) coconut palm sugar over the butter.
3.   Arrange pineapple slices to fit nicely into the bottom of the buttered glass baking dish. Add pecans placing one into the center of each opening in the pineapple and one on each side.
4.   Put beans and 3 eggs in blender. Blend on high, scraping sides occasionally, until beans are pureed and mixture is smooth.
5.   Combine remaining eggs, coconut oil, and vanilla extract in a small bowl. Add to blender and blend until smooth, scraping sides occasionally.
6.   Add egg mixture to blender. Blend on high, scraping sides of blender as needed until well combined.
7.   Combine 1/3 cup (80 mL) coconut palm sugar, coconut flour, baking powder, and baking soda in another small bowl, mixing thoroughly. Add to blender, blending until smooth.
8.   Add sugar mixture to blender. Blend on high, scraping sides often until well combined.

9.   Gently pour batter into glass baking dish on top of pineapple and pecans.
10.   Bake for about 45 minutes, until lightly golden around the edges and a knife inserted into the center comes out clean.
11.   Cool on a cloth covered rack.
12.   When cool, place a serving plate face down on top of the cake. While firmly holding both sides of the baking dish and serving plate flip them over and allow the cake to slide out of the baking dish onto the serving plate.
13.   Top each slice with a tsp. (5 mL) of sugar-free whipped topping, if desired.

CHOCOLATE BLACK BEAN CAKE

YIELD: Serves 10
Per portion:

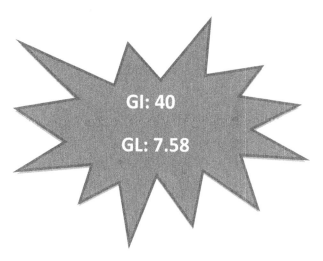

GI: 40
GL: 7.58

CALORIES: 226; Carbohydrates: 18.96g; Fiber: 3.56g; Protein: 7.21g; Fat: 14.44g; Saturated Fats: 8.57g; Sodium: 254.28mg

INGREDIENTS:
- 16 oz. (454 g) cooked black beans, at room temperature
- 5 large eggs
- ½ cup (120 mL) coconut palm sugar
- 3 Tbsp. (44 mL) coconut oil
- 3 Tbsp. (44 mL) organic unsalted butter, at room temperature
- 6 Tbsp. (89 mL) unsweetened cocoa powder
- 1 Tbsp. (15 mL) unsweetened cocoa powder
- 1 Tbsp. (15 mL) dry instant coffee crystals

- 1 tsp. (5 mL) vanilla extract
- 1 tsp. (5 mL) almond extract
- 1 Tbsp. (15 mL) extra virgin olive oil
- 1 tsp. (5 mL) aluminum-free baking powder
- ½ tsp. (2 mL) baking soda
- ½ tsp. (2 mL) sea salt
- 10 fresh strawberries, rinsed and gently patted dry

FOR FROSTING:
- 5 oz. (237 mL) Neufchatel cheese, at room temperature
- 2 Tbsp. (39 mL) cocoa
- 1 or 2 drops liquid stevia to taste, if desired
- One 3 1/2 oz. (104 mL) chocolate bar, 85% cocoa
- 1 Tbsp. (15 mL) unsalted, organic butter

PREPARATION:
1. Preheat oven to 325° F (163° C).
2. Spread olive oil over cooking surface of two 9 X 2 inch (23 X 4 cm) round glass baking dishes, and sprinkle surfaces with 1 Tbsp. (15 mL) cocoa powder. Set aside.
3. Put beans (if you use canned beans, drain them first) and 3 eggs in blender. Blend on high, scraping sides occasionally, until beans are pureed and mixture is completely smooth.
4. Combine remaining 2 eggs, coconut oil, butter, almond and vanilla extracts in a small bowl.
5. Add egg mixture to blender. Blend on high, scraping sides of blender as needed until very well combined.
6. Combine sugar, remaining cocoa powder, baking powder, baking soda, and instant

coffee crystals in another small bowl, mixing thoroughly.

7.   Add sugar mixture to blender. Blend on high, scraping sides often until well combined and creamy smooth.

8.   Pour equally into cocoa sprinkled baking dishes and bake for about 30 minutes, or until knife inserted in center of cake comes out clean.

9.   Remove glass baking dishes to a cloth covered wire rack to cool.

10. Turn one cake onto a serving platte, forming the bottom layer of your creation. (You can do this as you did in the Pina Colada Up-side-down cake, if it feels safer....)

11. Prepare the frosting: In a small mixing bowl, using an electric mixer, beat Neufchatel cheese, butter, 2 Tbsp. (30 mL) cocoa, and stevia to taste.

12. Spread a small amount of the frosting on the top of the bottom layer.

13. Turn second cake from its baking dish onto a serving plate, and turn it once again onto the top of the first cake, placing it with its top side up.

14. Frost the sides and then the top of the cake.

15. When ready to serve, melt chocolate over double boiler and drizzle 1 tsp. (5 mL) on each of 10 slices.

16. Garnish each slice with a lovely fresh strawberry.

CHOCOLATE RASPBERRY GANACHE CUPCAKES

YIELD: Serves 12
Per portion:

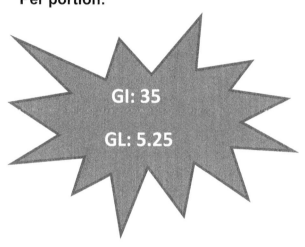

GI: 35

GL: 5.25

CALORIES: 126.45; Carbohydrates: 15g; Fiber: 2.56g; Protein: 5g; Fat: 12g; Saturated Fats: 3.15g; Sodium: 114mg

INGREDIENTS:
- One 16 oz. (454 g) can large butter beans, drained
- 6 eggs
- 1/4 cup (60 mL) coconut oil, melted
- 1/3 cup (80 mL) coconut palm sugar
- 1/3 cup (80mL) coconut flour
- 1 ½ tsp. (7 mL) aluminum free baking powder
- 1 tsp. (5 mL) baking soda
- 1 tsp. (5 mL) organic vanilla extract
- 1 tsp. (5 mL) organic almond extract

- **FILLING AND FROSTING:**
- 12 tsp. (59 mL) 100% pure fruit raspberry jam
- One 3 1/2 oz. (104 mL) chocolate bar, 85% cocoa
- 1 Tbsp. (15 mL) unsalted organic butter
- 2 Tbsp. (30 mL) Unsweetened almond milk

PREPARATION:
1. Preheat oven to 325° F (163° C).
2. Put 12 cupcake papers in cupcake baking tin.
3. Put beans and 3 eggs in blender. Blend on high, scraping sides occasionally, until beans are pureed and mixture is very smooth and creamy.
4. Combine remaining eggs, coconut oil, vanilla and almond extract in a small bowl.
5. Add egg mixture to blender. Blend on high, scraping sides of blender as needed until well combined.
6. Combine sugar, baking powder, and baking soda in another small bowl, mixing thoroughly.
7. Add sugar mixture to blender. Blend on high, scraping sides often until well combined.
8. Spoon mixture evenly into 12 cupcake papers.
9. Bake for about 25 minutes, until lightly golden around the edges and wooden pick inserted in center of middle cupcake comes out clean.
10. When cupcakes are cool, fill each cupcake with 1 tsp. (5 mL) of sugar-free raspberry jam.
11. Melt chocolate bar in top of double boiler. Add butter and almond milk, stirring to combine thoroughly.
12. Top each cupcake with 1 tsp. (5 mL) of hot, melted chocolate.

Are You Sweet Enough Already?

ANGEL FOOD CAKE WITH CHOCOLATE WHIPPED CREAM FROSTING AND DARK CHOCOLATE DRIZZLE

YIELD: 12 servings
Per portion:

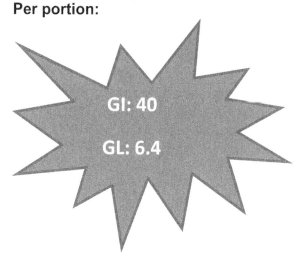

GI: 40

GL: 6.4

CALORIES: 142; Carbohydrates: 6.12g; Fiber: 2.13g; Protein: 9.10g; Fat: 9g; Saturated Fats: 5g; Sodium: 122.86mg

INGREDIENTS FOR CAKE:
- 2 cups (480 mL) liquid egg whites (about 12 egg whites)
- ¼ cup (60 mL) vanilla egg based unsweetened protein powder
- ¼ cup (60 mL) almond meal flour, twice sifted
- 3 Tbsp. (44 mL) powdered egg whites
- 8 packets stevia
- 1 Tbsp. (15 mL) unsalted organic butter
- 1 tsp. (5 mL) organic vanilla extract

- 1 tsp. (5 mL) organic almond extract
- 1 tsp. (5 mL) cream of tarter
- 1 tsp. (5 mL) xanthan gum
- ¼ tsp. (1 mL) baking powder

INGREDIENTS FOR FROSTING:
- 1 cup (240 mL) heavy cream (chilled)
- 2 Tbsp. (30 mL) unsweetened cocoa powder
- 2 packets stevia
- 1 Tbsp. (15 mL) cold water
- ½ tsp. (2 mL) unflavored gelatin powder
- ½ tsp. (2 mL) organic vanilla extract
- ½ tsp. (2 mL) organic almond extract
- One 85% dark chocolate bar (3 1/2 oz.) (104 mL) for drizzle

PREPARATION:

For Cake:
1. Heat oven to 350° F (177° C).
2. Coat the insides of a Bundt pan with butter, especially in the bottom and on the deep insides.
3. In a very clean (free of any oil residues – this is important) mixing bowl, combine the egg whites, stevia, cream of tartar, xanthan gum, baking powder, vanilla and almond extract.
4. Beat on low setting to combine, then beat on high until very stiff peaks form, for about four minutes.
5. In a small bowl, sift together protein powder, powdered egg whites, and twice sifted almond flour. Sift again.

6. Sprinkle half the protein powder over the egg white mixture. Mix at low speed to combine.
7. Add the remaining dry ingredient mixture to the egg white mixture, and mix on low for a few more seconds just to combine thoroughly.
8. Beat on high setting for 6 seconds.
9. With a very clean bowl scraper (being sure that there is no oil residue) fold the mixture together a few times.
10. Place about half the mixture in the Bundt pan smoothing the top with your clean bowl scraper. Tap the pan on the counter a few times to release a few bubbles, then add the rest of the batter to your Bundt pan. Tap the pan a few more times on the counter.
11. Bake for about 35 minutes, or until wooden toothpick comes out clean.
12. Remove from oven, place serving plate over cake in Bundt pan. While holding sides of pan and plate securely, flip them over to allow cake to slide out of pan and onto serving plate.
13. When the cake has cooled to room temperature, prepare the frosting.

For Frosting:
1. In a small heat-proof bowl, add the cold water and sprinkle the gelatin on top. Let stand for 4 minutes.
2. Bring a small amount of water to a boil in a small saucepan, and place the small bowl of gelatin and water in the saucepan and allow it

to simmer gently until the gelatin has dissolved completely – about five minutes.

3. Remove the bowl of gelatin mixture when fully dissolved, and allow it to cool to room temperature.

4. In a medium sized mixing bowl, beat the cream, vanilla and almond extract, cocoa powder, and stevia until soft peaks begin to form, scraping sides often with a clean bowl scraper.

5. Add the cooled gelatin mixture and beat just until stiff peaks begin to form. (Don't beat too long or you will have butter!)

6. Slice the cake in half horizontally.

7. Using about one third of the frosting, frost the top of the bottom half of the cake.

8. Place the top half of the cake back on top, and spread the remaining two thirds of frosting over the top and sides of the cake.

9. Melt the chocolate bar in a small heat resistant bowl over very hot water.

10. Drizzle the melted chocolate over the top of the cake, allowing some chocolate to flow over the sides of the cake.

Are You Sweet Enough Already?

SPECIAL BONUS SECTION

GLYCEMIC INDEX AND GLYCEMIC LOAD

The development of the Glycemic Index was an awesome beginning, (it's a ranking of the blood sugar raising potentials of carbohydrate foods.) But even low glycemic sources of carbohydrates can spike blood sugar levels if you eat too much of them. As my Grammy would say, "A slice is nice, but a slab will turn you into a slob."

Research has been ongoing into the causes of all the confusion. This is not surprising after witnessing that it took 30 years to recognize that fat was not the culprit causing heart disease, obesity, hypertension, and related diseases.

Then, recently, in 2013, a precedent setting meeting of international nutrition experts convened in Stresa, Italy. The outcome of their meeting was a consensus statement proclaiming that "The Glycemic Load (GL) is the single best predictor of the glycemic response."

Members of this committee included the developer of the glycemic load (GL), Dr. Walter Willett, and the chair of Epidemiology at Harvard's School of Public Health and the inventors of the Glycemic Index, Drs. David Jenkins and Thomas Wolever of the University of Toronto.

The Consensus Committee adjourned their summit meeting with the following statement: "Convincing scientific evidence confirms low glycemic load eating reduces out-of-control blood sugar levels lowering risks from:

- Obesity and Coronary Heart Disease
- Diabetes and Prediabetes
- Related diseases (co-morbidities) including hypertension"

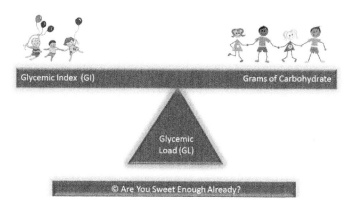

The Basis of Low Glycemic Eating Rests Squarely Upon the *Glycemic Load (GL)*

When you boil it all down, you see that the truth is that effective blood sugar control has its basis in low glycemic eating and the basis of low glycemic eating rests squarely upon the glycemic load.

Yet, even after the above nutrition proclamation, do you see the glycemic index and glycemic load scores included among the "Nutrition Facts" listed on the packaging of any manufactured food-like products in the U.S.? No, you do not.

35

Meals that contain high glycemic carbohydrates automatically fuel sugar addiction. That's because high glycemic carbohydrates rapidly convert to glucose (sugar) during digestion. This is why your blood sugar surges so high and fast. And if you don't burn it off right away, it is stored as fat.

Over time, consistent high blood sugar levels lead to fat storage and insulin resistance. That sets the perfect stage for obesity and diabetes. Maybe you are there already, and feel helpless, but you're not.

In this section you will learn how to use the Glycemic Index (GI) and Glycemic Load (GL) to select carbohydrates and build recipes.

You have seen some recipes and know that there are desserts that do not skyrocket your blood sugar levels. You don't have to deal with crashing down from a sugar high after a few moments of pleasure anymore.

No, they don't contain any of the usual culprits such as table sugar, high fructose corn syrup, or any of the other sugar-derived sweeteners.... And they don't contain any chemically produced sweeteners like saccharin, aspartame, or Splenda, either. (None of those thieves are your friends!)

There are better ingredients you can use to build delicious desserts that create health and are easy to prepare. They will satisfy your sweet tooth and quell your cravings. Now you can walk away from sugar addiction savoring … a little slice of heaven.

HARVESTING THE POWER OF THE GLYCEMIC INDEX:

3 SIMPLE STEPS TO SELECT THE BEST CARBOHYDRATE INGREDIENTS

There are three factors to consider when you are designing a recipe for blood sugar control: the Glycemic Index, the number of carbs, and the Glycemic Load.

Choosing carbohydrates with a Low Glycemic Index (0 – 55) is always best. (Below you will find links to excellent resources that will give you the numbers you need for all of your calculations.)

#1. The Glycemic Index Ranges from Low to High:

0 - 55   Low

56 - 69   Medium

70 +   High

The first step is to determine the glycemic index of your carbohydrate ingredients.

You will find extensive Glycemic Index scores at ***The National Institutes of Health***[1] which offers two supplemental table PDF's you can download and save on your computer.

One PDF includes test results on individuals with impaired glucose tolerance. The other has results on those with normal glucose tolerance -- for a total of 2,480 entries. This is where you can locate the Glycemic Index of your ingredients. This is a free resource.

You may find that some ingredients are unlisted among the two National Institutes of Health PDF databases. That is because some ingredients have assigned values. Here are the assigned values for unlisted ingredients:

Unlisted Dairy Products	30
Unlisted Vegetables	40
Unlisted fruits (botanically, fruits are part of the vegetable family)	40
Wheat flour products	70

#2. Knowing the carbohydrate content of your ingredients is the next step. Carb content can vary

---

[1] https://www.ncbi.nlm.nih.gov/pmc/articles/PMC2584181/bin/dc08-1239_index.html

wildly among similar ingredients, and the easiest way to get the bottom line is to add up all the carbs in all your ingredients to get the total carbs in your recipe.

Then you divide that total by the number of servings your recipe will provide.

The USDA National Nutrient Database for Standard Reference[2] provides very detailed nutrition information including carb counts based on portion sizes for over 8,000 foods. It is a free resource, too.

#3. The Glycemic Load Ranges from Low to High:

0 - 10   **Low**

11 -19   **Medium**

20 +   **High**

Keeping a Low Glycemic Load (0 -10) is always best.

When you have located the ingredient with the highest Glycemic Index, and the total amount of carbs for each serving of your recipe, you have what you need to calculate the Glycemic Load.

A simple grid is an easy way to keep track of the nutrition of your ingredients. It is a handy way to calculate the total amount of carbs (and any other nutrient you are keeping an eye on) in each serving.

---

[2] https://ndb.nal.usda.gov/ndb/

BUILDING A GRID TO KEEP THE SCORE

When you locate your nutrition information, it is easy to plug it into a grid as you go along. You may want to return to your grid and update if you decide to change a recipe at a later date. Excel is a wonderful program for this, but a pen and paper will work just fine. If you decide to use a pen and paper, a ruler might come in handy to keep things neat, especially if you are working with a recipe with a long list of ingredients.

Here is a simple nutrition grid built in Excel for our *Chocolate Avocado Cream Pie*:

Chocolate Avocado Cream Pie Nutrition							
Ingredient	Cal	Carbs	Fiber	Fat	Sat Fat	Protein	Sodium
1 cup ground pecans	1588	31.44	21.6	163.2	14	80	0
1/2 cup almond meal	213	8	4	18.66	1.33	8	0
1/2 cup flax meal	600	32	32	48	4	20	32
2 Tbsp. cocoa	24	6.16	3.6	1.48	0.88	2	0
2 packets of stevia	0	2	0	0	0	0	0
2 Tbsp. coconut oil	234	0	6	26.32	23.48	0	0
1 Tbsp. butter	102	0	0	11.52	7.29	0.12	2
5 large avacodos (2 cups)	736	39.24	30.8	67.49	9.8	9.2	32
6 Tbsp. cocoa	72	18.48	10.8	4.44	2.64	6	0
9 packets of stevia	0	9	0	0	0	0	0
2 Tbsp. coffee crystals	98	20	0	0	0	4	10
1 cup fresh bing cherries	87	22	3	0	0	1	0
---Serving 12	3754	188.32	111.8	341.1	63.42	130.32	76
------ per serving	312.83	15.69	9.32	28.43	5.29	10.86	6.33

WORKING WITH YOUR GRID:
List all of your *ingredients* and their amounts along the left side, as in the above illustration. Next, list the specific *nutrients* you'd like to keep track of along the top.

Now, plug in the nutrition information from the USDA Database into the columns for each ingredient used in the recipe. For instance, if your recipe contains 2 cups of an ingredient, you research the nutritive values for 2 cups, and plug those values into your grid.

Create columns for any nutrients you would like to keep track of. When you have finished inputting the nutrition values for the amount of each ingredient, you sum or add up each column from top to bottom. This way you know the calories, carbs, fiber, fat, saturated fat, protein, sodium, and any other nutrient you want to keep an eye on in the entire recipe.

Time Saving Tip: You might want to *calculate the carbs per serving* first, so that you can alter the ingredient list as you are building your recipe if necessary. (Add up total carbs in recipe ÷ divide by number of servings.)

After you add up each column, divide the column totals by the number of servings your recipe will provide. That will be the amount of each nutrient per serving. Now you are ready to calculate the glycemic load.

QUICK & EASY GUIDE TO CALCULATING THE GLYCEMIC LOAD

When you arrive at the total carbohydrate content per serving, you can determine the Glycemic Load of your recipe.

Select the carbohydrate ingredient in your recipe with the highest Glycemic Index (GI). Multiply the GI of that ingredient by the grams of carbs in a serving. Divide your result by 100. Now you have the Glycemic Load (GL) for one serving.

Highest GI Ingredient X Grams of Carbohydrate per serving / 100 = GL

A TALE OF TWO PIES: FOOD FOR THOUGHT

In the above *Chocolate Avocado Cream Pie* Nutrition chart, the ingredient with the highest glycemic index is the Bing Cherries with a glycemic index of 40.

With a glycemic index of 40 and 15.69 grams of carbs per serving, the glycemic load is 6.28 per each of 12 servings. (Example: 40 X 15.69 = 627.6 / 100 = 6.28.)

If you selected strawberries with a glycemic index of 40 with 14.83 grams of carbs instead of cherries, the glycemic load per serving drops a bit to 5.93.

But what if you topped your pie with raspberries? There would be no glycemic index at all! Most of this dessert is fiber, monounsaturated fat, and protein!

HOW SWEET IT IS – COMPARING THE GI OF TABLE SUGAR (70) WITH LOW GLYCEMIC ALTERNATIVES:

Stevia	GI = 0
Xylitol	GI = 7
Coconut Palm Sugar	GI = 35
Blackstrap Molasses	GI = 55

Stevia is a plant that is very sweet. Stevia is available as a plant, in packets or a liquid which takes very little to sweeten a recipe.

Xylitol is another sweetening option you might consider. Xylitol is derived from North American hardwood. Xylitol is a great substitute for table sugar as it behaves like table sugar in a recipe, while it has a much lower glycemic index.

Coconut palm sugar comes from trees, too. Coconut palm sugar contains a handful of minerals and 16 amino acids, making it quite an improvement over brown sugar, again, with a much lower glycemic index. Both xylitol and coconut palm sugar can be used ounce for ounce to replace the sugar called for in a recipe.

Blackstrap molasses contains two handfuls of minerals, a low glycemic index, and the *Gingerbread Baby Cakes* would not be the same without it.

THE POWER IS NOW IN YOUR OWN HANDS

Don't just take my word for it, do your own research. You may be surprised at some of the results you find.

Between the National Institutes of Health Database, the USDA Nutrient Database for Standard Reference, and a simple grid to keep track of food values, you can build your own cookbook if you like.

As you have read through these recipes I hope you have discovered some simple substitutions that you can use to turn even your most beloved heirloom recipes into healthy desserts for yourself and your loved ones.

For a more detailed review of using the Glycemic Index and Glycemic Load to build your own recipes, see **Low Glycemic Happiness 120 Recipes for Blood Sugar Control** [3] available at Amazon.com and other booksellers in paperback and Kindle. This book also contains a treasure of research links to studies in *The Heart of the Matter.*

---

[3]
https://www.amazon.com/gp/bookseries/B017WCB7KK/ref=dp_st_15 23803991

Explore our blog at **LowGlycemicHappiness.com**[4] for more information and resources.

"Like" ***Low Glycemic Happiness on Facebook***[5] for more ideas and insights on current health issues.

---

[4] http://lowglycemichappiness.com/lgh-blog.html
[5] https://www.facebook.com/LowGlycemicHappiness

Are You Sweet Enough Already?

Are You Sweet Enough Already?

Are You Sweet Enough Already?

Printed in Great Britain
by Amazon

62495043R00037